Weight Watchers Freestyle Cookbook 2021

Easy, Healthy and Delicious WW Smart Points Recipes for Rapid Weight Loss & Heal Your Body

Bandle fougen

Table of Contents

Introduction

Weight Watchers Diet stands as one of the most unique dietary programs out there in the market. It is also regarded as the 4th most effective diet in several lists that rank the world's best diets.

First established by Jean Nidetch during the 1920s, the diet has taken the world by storm as of late, thanks to its unique approach to keeping your healthy, all the while allowing to lose weight without the need to sacrifice the food that you love.

Unlike most other diets out there, Weight Watchers does not specifically tell people what kind of food they should eat or what kind of meals they should prepare.

Instead, this diet encourages people to make healthier choices regarding food and increase their physical activity through a very intricately designed point system.

While there does exist a form a Weight Watchers Diet that includes no counting of points, we will not discuss that here.

How these diet works are by adding a specific amount of "Smart Points" to food and ingredients that ultimately allows you to keep your food intake under control and encourage you to a healthier lifestyle.

The Freestyle expansion, which was established in 2017, introduced almost 200 foods that are now considered "Zero" point food. So, the Freestyle essentially greatly expands the array of food you can consume without worrying about ruining your health!

This particular book is designed to give beginners a basic idea of how the whole program works.

Keeping that in mind, the first few pages of the book contain the basic information required to get you started with the weight watchers program. After that, you will have the chance to explore a plethora of amazing and heart-warming recipes.

So, what are you waiting for? Dive right in and enjoy the amazing world of Weight Watchers Freestyle!

Chapter 1: Weight Watcher Basics

The History of Weight Watchers

To fully appreciate the history and origin of the Weight Watchers Program, we must travel back to the year 1923, when a humble homemaker who went by the name Jean Nidetech took bold steps to help women lose weight and keep their food cravings under control came up with the amazing idea of Weight Watchers.

However, if you want to fully understand the depth of the discovery of this diet, you have to look at it from Jean's Perspective.

Curious to know why?

Well...

Jean herself was an individual who had constantly been suffering from obesity. After going through a lot of different diets, the Weight Watchers program was the one that allowed her to bring the food lust under control and trim down her fat.

However, during her journey, she did try out several different approaches to lose weight, including a few diets.

While these programs and diets helped her lose weight, she soon noticed that just as soon as she let go of the diet, she started gaining even more weight.

This led to an epiphany.

She soon realized that there are millions of people worldwide who are suffering from obesity, which inspired her to develop a solution that would help them reach their goals.

However, she soon realized that just dieting won't solve the obesity problem in the long run! The main problem that led to millions of people suffering from obesity worldwide was "Lack of Control."

Based on her Personal experience, It didn't really matter which diet you follow; it ultimately came down to a simple matter of control. If you cannot control your food intake, you will soon gain back all the weight that you lost.

Keeping that simple notion in mind, Jean took the initiative and created a health support group to help her friends and family members who were in need and were suffering from obesity and other diet problems.

This group eventually became the Weight Watchers organization.

The Weight Watchers program that we follow today, the "Freestyle Program," in our case, is the peak form of an idea that was laid way back in the 1920s!

The Weight Watchers Freestyle won't only help you to trim down your fat. Still, it will also improve your physical and psychological health.

What are Smart Points?

The Smart Points system is the program's beating heart, which essentially drives the diet.

Unlike most diets out there, though, Weight Watchers doesn't really ask you to follow a very strict dietary regime that would force you to eliminate all of your favorite food from your life!

Rather, this program encourages you to make healthy food and life choices by implementing an aura of the carefully crafted "Points" system that assigns a point to different ingredients/food.

This pointing system is further accompanied by a Physical Point system, but that is not our book's focus!

Smart Points are specific numerical values that are assigned to certain ingredients and food-based several different factors.

In general, The lower the Smart Point number of a certain ingredient, the better and healthier it is.

Weight Watchers doesn't impose a very strict dietary restriction on you. It will still give you a specified weekly Smart Points budget based on your target, sex, height, weight, and a few other factors.

The main idea is that you can consume as many foods as you want, just as long as you are not exceeding your allocated budget.

The next section explains how the Smart Points system works in detail.

How do Smart Points Work?

As you may have already guessed, the Weight Watchers program's beating heart is the "Smart Points" system itself.

So, let me break down the points system to you to give you a better understanding of the Science behind the program.

Keep in mind that the Freestyle program uses a revamped version of the "Smart Point" program. Therefore, I will explain the Smart Points system here.

A simple formula for calculating the Smart points of your meal is done using the formula below.

Points = (Calories + (Fat x 4) – (Fiber x 10))/50

However, if you want greater accuracy, you can always refer to the provided list of the common ingredients (and their SP) in the section below.

As for calculating your daily Smart Points limit, some fantastic calculators out there will help you achieve that. Two good examples are

http://www.healthyweightforum.org/eng/calculators/ww:points:allowed/

or

http://www.calculator.net/weight:watchers:points:calculator.html

To give you an idea, though, let us follow an example where we assume that you 20 years old male and have a weight of 70kgs with a height of 5 feet, and your target is to lose 10 kg, and then your allocated SP will be 30.

However, the best way to calculate your Daily and Weekly Allowance is still through the official Weight Watchers App provided upon availing of your membership.

But if you want to experiment with the program for free, then the websites mentioned above will help you, while the following apps will help you as well.

- Ultimate Food Diary App (This app is the only one that has been updated to provide services that resemble the Freestyle meal plan)
- Track Bites (This is yet another app that is very close to the official WW app. However, this did not support the Freestyle program at the time of writing but was supposed to be updated very soon)

This means that you can eat as much as you want as long as you are not crossing your daily point limit.

Pros and Cons of Freestyle

Like every other diet, Freestyle also comes with many health advantages and cons that you should consider.

- The Weight Watchers program won't impose horrible food restrictions upon you
- Through the membership and meeting, you will be able to receive various cooking advice and nutritional tips while sharing your own experience
- Even kids are allowed to join the experience!
- The Smart Points system encourages you to maintain your portions, which will allow you to gradually and steadily lose your weight
- Through Fit Points, exercise is largely encouraged, which helps to maintain an excellent physique
- Some people might not feel comfortable sharing their Personal information in group meetings
- Keeping track of your Smart Points all throughout the day might get tedious if you

don't have the patience

- Weekly weight loss progress might discourage you as the changes won't be that drastic initially

The freedom to eat might make it difficult for you to stay in control

Common Ingredients and Smart Points (Old)

Below is a list of the most common ingredients alongside their associated Smart Point for your convenience.

Food with 0 SP

- Coffee
- Banana
- Apple
- Strawberries
- Chicken Breast
- Salad
- Blueberries
- Grapes
- Tomatoes
- Watermelon
- Egg White
- Lettuce
- Deli Sliced Turkey Breast
- Baby Carrots
- Orange
- Cucumber
- Broccoli
- Water
- Green Beans
- Pineapple

- Corn On The Cob (medium)
- Cherries
- Cantaloupe
- Spinach
- Fresh Fruit
- Raspberries
- Shrimp
- Asparagus
- Celery
- Cherry Tomatoes
- Carrots
- Yogurt
- Peach
- Sweet Red Potatoes
- Pear
- Salsa
- Tuna
- Diet Coke
- Mushrooms
- Onions
- Black Beans
- Blackberries
- Zucchini
- Grape Tomatoes
- Mixed Berries
- Grapefruit
- Nectarine
- Mango
- Mustard

Food with 1 SP

- Sugar
- Almond Milk
- Egg
- Guacamole
- Half and Half
- Salad Dressing

Food with 2 SP

- Cream
- Avocado
- 1 Slice Of Bread
- Scrambled Egg with milk/ butter
- Luncheon Meat, deli-sliced, or ham (2 ounces)
- 2 t tablespoon of Hummus

Food with 3 SP

- Milk Skimmed
- 1 tablespoon of Mayonnaise
- Chocolate Chip Cookies
- Sweet potatoes ½ a cup
- 3 ounce of boneless Pork Chop
- 1 ounce of flour Tortilla
- Italian Salad Dressing 2 tablespoon
- 3 slices of cooked Turkey Bacon
- 1 cup of Cottage Cheese
- An ounce of crumbled feta

Food with 4 SP

- Olive Oil
- American Cheese 1 slice
- Low Fat Milk 1%, 1 Cup

- Cheddar Cheese 1 ounce
- Red Wine 5 ounce
- ¼ cup of Almond
- 5 ounce of White Wine
- Tortilla Chips 1 ounce
- Shredded Cheddar Cheese
- 1 tablespoon of honey
- 102 ounce of English Muffin
- Mashed Potatoes

Food with 5 SP

- Butter
- 3 Slices of Cooked Bacon
- Reduced Fat Milk 1 Cup
- Cooked Oatmeal 1 cup
- Plain Baked Potato, 6 ounce
- Regular Beer, 12 ounce
- 1 cup of cooked regular/ whole wheat pasta
- Hamburger Bun
- Ranch Salad Dressing
- Any type of Bagel (2 ounces)
- 1 cup of Spaghetti

Food With 6+ SP

- White Rice (6)
- Brown Rice (6)
- Peanut Butter 2 tablespoon (6)
- 1 Whole Cup Of Milk (7)
- 20 ounce of French Fries (13)
- 1 cup of cooked Quinoa (6)

Freestyle Updated Zero Point Ingredients

- Peas such as chickpeas, sugar snap peas, black-eyed, etc.
- Beans such as black beans, kidney beans, pinto beans, fat-free refried beans, soybeans, sprouts, etc.
- Lentils
- Corn such as baby corn, sweet corn, corn on the cob
- Skinless Chicken Breast
- Skinless Turkey Breast
- Tofu
- Egg and Egg Whites
- Fish and Shellfish
- Yogurt
- Lean Ground Beef
- Non-Fat and Plain Greek Yogurt
- All Fruits
- All Vegetables

To give you a more detailed look at the list, the following now hold a 0 Smart Point value.

- Yogurt
- Plain Yogurt
- Greek Yogurt
- Watermelon
- Watercress
- Water Chestnuts
- Stir-Fried Vegetables
- Mixed Vegetables
- Sticks of Vegetables
- Turnips
- Turkey Breast
- Turkey Breast Tenderloin

- Ground Turkey Breast
- Tomato
- Tomato Sauce
- Tofu
- Taro
- Tangerine
- Tangelo
- Star fruit
- Winter and Summer Squash
- Spinach
- Shellfish
- Shallots
- Scallions
- Sauerkraut
- Chicken satay
- Sashimi
- Salsa
- Salad
- Lentils
- Lime
- Lettuce
- Litchi
- Mangoes
- Mung Dal
- Mushroom Caps
- Nectarine
- Okra
- Onions
- Orange
- Parsley
- Pea Shoot

- Peaches
- Pear
- Pepper
- Pickles
- Pineapple
- Plums
- Pomegranate Seeds
- Pomelo
- Pumpkin
- Pumpkin Puree
- Radish
- Salad Mixed Greens
- Salad Three Bean
- Lemon Zest
- Leek
- Kiwifruit
- Jicama
- Jerk Chicken Breast
- Jackfruit
- Heart of Palm
- Guava
- Mixed Baby Greens
- Ginger Root
- Grape Fruit
- Fruit Cup
- Fruit Cocktail
- Fish Fillet
- Fruit
- Fish
- Figs
- Fennel

- Escarole
- Endive
- Egg Whites
- Eggs
- Apples
- Arrowroot
- Applesauce
- Artichoke
- Artichoke Hearts
- Bamboo Shoots
- Banana
- Beans
- Beets
- Blueberries
- Blackberries
- Broccoli
- Brussels
- Cabbage
- Carrots
- Cauliflower
- Cherries
- Chicken Breast
- Clementine
- Cucumber
- Dragon Fruit
- Egg Substitute
- Dates

And a few more.

Chapter 2: Success Tips for Weight Watchers Freestyle

Below are some amazing tips that will help you during the early days of your Weight Watchers Journey.

- Make sure to learn how to maintain and control your portions. Having a good understanding of standard measurements such as ounce, cups, etc. is crucial when creating a meal plan. You don't want to overshoot your meal portions, as it might lead to an unsatisfactory result.
- Although the Smart Points for the recipes is roughly calculated in this book using the provided outline (in the appendix), it is still recommended that you learn how to figure the Smart Points by yourself.
- Make sure to skip "Diet" soft drinks. While they might be free from unwanted calories, they still pack a good load of artificial sweeteners, leading to various medical issues.
- While practicing your portion control, you should never skip on exercise! Even if it is for 5-10 minutes, you should try not to avoid a short daily exercise routine.
- When you are eating, always try to split the meals if you have someone else to share your meals. This will allow you to lower down both your calorie and point intake.
- Using the SP list found in the end, experiment with various ingredients and recipes using this book as a source of inspiration and create your very own meals!

Chapter 3: FAQs

Freestyle Exclusive Changes

When considering the Freestyle Points System, there are a few crucial things that you should keep in mind.

- The new "Zero" Point foods

As you may have already understood, this isPerhaps the biggest change to the Weight Watchers program. Various food items that previously had a significant number of points have been completely cut down to "Zero" points that make the diet much more versatile when choosing your meals and creating your plan.

- About Smart Points

The updated Freestyle program will still use the same method of calculation. However, your daily SmartPoint allocation will change a bit to balance out the new foods that are all zeroed out now. Suppose you are already a member of the Weight Watchers program. In that case, you may be able to do this through their designated app. Alternatively, you may use the apps mentioned in the previous section.

- Weekly Point Allowance

Despite having a change in your daily point allowance, the weekly allowance will still remain the same. This means that you will be able to include more food and adjust your plans with greater flexibility.

- Rollover Points

This is yet another feature that is exclusive to the new program. The Rollover point system allows you to carry over a maximum of 4 SmartPoints to the coming week. For example, assuming that you have a weekly limit of 120 Smart Points, if you use 116 points in the previous week, you will have a SmartPoint allocation of 124 points for the latter week. This is a good strategy to follow if you have any major upcoming events.

With that, the basics are pretty much covered, and you are now ready to explore the recipes themselves!

Keep in mind that there is a list of food items at the end of the book. I have illustrated several common ingredients and food groups alongside their SP points.

Understanding the Cost of the Diet

Since the diet does not specifically bind you to a fixed diet plan, you are free to choose the recipes and ingredients you can use, allowing you to carve out your meal plans according to your Personal budget.

However, suppose you are looking for an online membership or are interested in joining the meetings. In that case, you are to pay a very small signup fee.

At the time of writing, the online membership had a fee of 17.5$Per month, which had an additional 29.95$ initiation fee.

On the other hand, you can also go for In-Person meetings with unlimited access for $39.95, which has its Perks.

So, forgetting the Weight Watchers community's official support, you may expect a bill of 50:60$.

Keep in mind that these numbers are subject to change, and it is highly recommended that visit

www.weightwatchers.com to get an updated value of their current plans.

But everything said and done, the plan ultimately depends on you!

The only thing to keep in mind is to "not" cross your daily Smart Point limit.

In terms of following the Freestyle Diet, the most important thing to remember is to not exceed your weekly allocated Smart Points limit.

Can Weight Watchers Help with Weight Loss?

Perhaps this is the main reason why you are even reading this book, right?

Well, the idea behind losing weight through the Weight Watchers Freestyle Diet isn't as straightforward as it may seem!

Mainly because the core aim of this diet is to not only act as a means of "Losing Excess Fat" but also as a means to "Keep You Under Control" in the long run.

This program is not designed to be a temporary solution but rather a long-term process that helps you to stay fit and lean for the rest of your journey.

In one of the previous sections, I have already explained the basic concepts of "HOW" you can calculate your weekly allocated Smart Points limit.

Since this weekly limit largely depends on multiple parameters such as your current weight, target weight, time, age, sex, etc. the weekly Smart Point limit largely varies from Person to Person, so there's no "One" answer as to how much weight you can lose within a week.

It will ultimately depend on how much effort you are willing to put into the diet and how strictly you will follow it.

However, if you move at a good pace and adhere to your allocated Smart Points limit, you will quickly trim down 1-2 pounds of unwanted fat each week!

And the best part?

As long as you are sticking to the program, those unwanted and lost fats won't even come back, thanks to the carefully thought out system!

Chapter 4: Breakfast Recipes

Ricotta Tomato and Egg Bread

Serving: 4
Prep Time: 5 minutes
Cook Time: 10 minutes

<u>Ingredients</u>

- 4 medium raw whole eggs
- 4 tablespoon of skimmed milk
- 4 slices of whole meal bread
- 4 sprays cooking spray
- 9 ounce of cherry tomatoes
- 9 ounce Ricotta cheese

<u>How To</u>

1. Lightly beat eggs and milk and season with black pepper
2. Take a shallow dish and add bread in layer
3. Pour egg mixture over and turn the bread several time to coat
4. Take a large-sized nonstick frying pan and place it over medium heat
5. Mist with cooking spray
6. Fry the bread in batches for about 2:3 minutes on each side until golden
7. Cut the slices in half and keep them on the side
8. Add tomatoes to the pan and stir for 2:3 minutes
9. Serve the bread with tomatoes and ricotta
10. Enjoy!

<u>Nutrition Values (Per Serving)</u>

- Calories: 254
- Fat: 9g
- Carbohydrates: 34g
- Protein: 8g

Berry Packed Granola Bowl

Serving: 6
Prep Time: 5 minutes
Cook Time: 25 minutes

Ingredients

- 1 ounce of Porridge oats
- 2 teaspoon of Maple Syrup
- Cooking spray as needed
- 4 medium Bananas
- 4 pots of Caramel Layered Fromage Frais
- 5 ounce of Fresh Fruit Salad such as strawberries, blueberries, and raspberries
- ¼ ounce of pumpkin seeds
- ¼ ounce of sunflower seeds
- ¼ ounce of dry Chia seeds
- ¼ ounce of Desiccated coconut

How To

1. Preheat your oven to 302 degrees Fahrenheit
2. Line up a baking tray with baking paper
3. Take a large bowl and add oats, seeds, maple syrup
4. Spread the mixture out on the baking tray
5. Mix with coconut oil spray and bake for 20 minutes, making sure to keep stirring it from time to time
6. Sprinkle coconut at the 15 minutes point
7. Remove from the oven and spread out on a cold baking tray
8. Slice bananas and layer in a bowl with Fromage Frais
9. Sprinkle granola on top and serve with the berries
10. Enjoy!

Nutrition Values (Per Serving)

- Calories: 446
- Fat: 29g
- Carbohydrates: 37g
- Protein: 13g

Lovely Chocolate Quinoa Bowl

Serving: 2
Prep Time: 10 minutes
Cook Time: 30 minutes

Ingredients

- 1 cup quinoa
- 1 cup almond milk, unsweetened
- 1 teaspoon cinnamon
- 1 banana
- 1 cup of water
- 2-3 tablespoons cocoa powder, unsweetened
- 2 tablespoons almond butter
- 1 tablespoon chia seeds, ground
- 2 tablespoons walnuts, optional
- ¼ cup raspberries, fresh

How To

1. Add cinnamon, milk, water, quinoa in a pot
2. Bring the mix to a boil before turning it down to low, let it simmer for 25-35 minutes, covered
3. Puree banana and add almond butter, flaxseed, cocoa powder
4. Scoop cup of quinoa into a bowl, top with pudding, raspberries, and walnuts
5. Serve and enjoy!

Nutrition (Per Serving)

- Calories: 390
- Fat: 20g
- Carbohydrates: 50g
- Protein: 12g

Refreshing Strawberry and Almond Smoothie

Serving: 2
Prep Time: 10 minutes
Cook Time: Nil

Ingredients

- 16 ounces unsweetened almond milk, vanilla
- 1 teaspoon natural sweetener such as Maple Syrup
- 4 ounces almond cream
- 1 scoop vanilla whey protein
- ¼ cup frozen strawberries, unsweetened

How To

1. Add listed ingredients to a blender
2. Blend until you have a smooth and creamy texture
3. Serve chilled and enjoy!

Nutrition (Per Serving)

- Calories: 304
- Fat: 25g
- Carbohydrates: 7g
- Protein: 15g

Lemon and Thyme Couscous Meal

Serving: 4
Prep Time: 5 minutes
Cook Time: 5 minutes

Ingredients

- 2 and ¾ cups vegetable stock
- Juice and zest of 1 lemon
- 2 tablespoons fresh thyme, chopped
- ¼ cup fresh parsley, chopped
- Salt and pepper for taste

How To

1. Take a pot and add the stock, lemon juice, thyme and boil
2. Stir in couscous and cover; remove heat
3. Let it sit for 5 minutes, fluff with a fork
4. Stir in lemon zest and parsley, season with salt and pepper
5. Enjoy!

Nutrition (Per Serving)

- Calories: 190
- Fat: 16g
- Carbohydrates: 12g
- Protein: 3g

Premium Zucchini Boats

Serving: 4
Prep Time: 10 minutes
Cook Time: 25 minutes

Ingredients

- 4 medium zucchinis
- ½ cup marinara sauce
- ¼ red onion, sliced
- ¼ cup kalamata olives, chopped
- ½ cup cherry tomatoes, sliced
- 2 tablespoons fresh basil

How To

1. Preheat your oven to 400 degrees Fahrenheit
2. Cut the zucchini half-lengthwise and shape them into boats
3. Take a bowl and add tomato sauce, spread 1 layer of sauce on top of each of the boat
4. Top with onion, olives, and tomatoes
5. Bake for 20-25 minutes
6. Top with basil and enjoy!

Nutrition (Per Serving)

- Calories: 278
- Fat: 20g
- Carbohydrates: 10g
- Protein: 15g

Almond Pancakes

Number of Servings: 6
Prep Time: 10 minutes
Cooking Time: 10 minutes

Ingredients

- 6 whole eggs
- ¼ cup almonds, toasted
- 2 ounces cocoa chocolate
- 1/3 cup coconut, shredded
- 1 teaspoon almond extract
- ½ teaspoon baking powder
- ¼ cup of coconut oil
- ¼ cup stevia
- 1 cup almond milk
- Cooking spray as needed
- Pinch of salt

How To

1. Take a bowl and add coconut flour, stevia, salt, baking powder, coconut and gently stir
2. Add coconut oil, eggs, almond milk, almond extract and stir well
3. Add chocolate, almond and whisk well
4. Take a pan and place it over medium heat, add 2 tablespoons batter, spread into a circle
5. Cook until golden and flip, transfer to pan
6. Repeat with remaining batter
7. Serve and enjoy!

Nutritional Values (Per Serving)

- Calories: 266

- Fat: 13g
- Carbohydrates: 10 g
- Protein: 11 g

Apple and Cinnamon Oatmeal

Serving: 2
Prep Time: 10 minutes
Cook Time: 10 minutes

Ingredients

- 1 and ¼ cups apple cider
- 1 apple, peeled, cored, and chopped
- 2/3 cups rolled oats
- 1 teaspoon ground cinnamon
- 1 tablespoon pure maple syrup

How To

1. Take a medium-sized saucepan, bring apple cider to boil over medium-high heat
2. Stir in apples, oats, cinnamon
3. Bring cereal to a boil and reduce heat to lower, simmer for 3-4 minutes until thickened
4. Spoon between two bowls and serve with maple syrup, enjoy!

Nutrition (Per Serving)

- Calories: 339
- Fat: 14g
- Carbohydrates: 40g
- Protein: 8g

Early Morning French Toast

Serving: 4
Prep Time: 15 minutes
Cook Time: 10 minutes

Ingredients

- 3 bananas, ripe
- 1 cup unsweetened almond milk
- Zest of 1 orange
- 1 teaspoon ground cinnamon
- ¼ teaspoon nutmeg, grated
- 4 French bread slices
- 1 tablespoon coconut oil

How To

1. Take a blender and add banana, milk, orange juice, zest, cinnamon, and nutmeg; blend well until smooth
2. Pour mixture into 9 by 13-inch baking dish, soak bread in mixture for 5 minutes each side
3. While the bread soaks, heat griddle over medium heat and melt coconut oil, swirl well to coat
4. Cook bread slices until golden brown, 5 minutes on each side
5. Serve and enjoy!

Nutrition (Per Serving)

- Calories: 200
- Fat: 12g
- Carbohydrates: 20g
- Protein: 6g

Awesome Pineapple Oatmeal

Serving: 5
Prep Time: 10 minutes
Cook Time: 4-8 hours

Ingredients

- 1 cup steel-cut oats
- 4 cups unsweetened almond milk
- 2 medium apples, slashed
- 1 teaspoon coconut oil
- 1 teaspoon cinnamon
- ¼ teaspoon nutmeg
- 2 tablespoons maple syrup
- A drizzle of lemon juice

Directions

1. Add listed ingredients to a cooking pan and mix well
2. Cook on very low flame for 8 hours/ or on high flame for 4 hours
3. Gently stir
4. Add toppings your desired toppings
5. Serve and enjoy!
6. Store in the fridge for later use; make sure to add a splash of almond milk after re-heating for added flavor

Nutrition Values (Per Serving)

- Calories: 180
- Fat: 5g
- Carbohydrates: 31g
- Protein: 5g

Awesome Breakfast Parfait

Serving: 2
Prep Time: 5 minutes
Cook Time: Nil

Ingredients

- 1 teaspoon salt
- ½ cup low-fat milk
- 1 cup all-purpose flour
- 1 teaspoon vanilla
- 4 beaten eggs
- 1 teaspoon baking soda
- 2 cups non-fat Greek Yogurt

Directions

1. Break up pretzels into small-sized portions and slice up the strawberries
2. Add Yogurt to the bottom of the glass and top with pretzels pieces and strawberries
3. Add more Yogurt and keep repeating until you have used up all ingredients
4. Enjoy!

Nutrition Values (Per Serving)

- Calorie: 304
- Fat: 1g
- Carbohydrates: 58g
- Protein: 15g

Nut Packed Porridge

Serving: 4
Prep Time: 10 minutes
Cook Time: 15 minutes

Ingredients

- 1 cup cashew nuts, raw and unsalted
- 1 cup pecan, halved
- 2 tablespoons stevia
- 4 teaspoons coconut oil, melted
- 2 cups of water

How To

1. Chop the nuts in a food processor and form a smooth paste
2. Add water, oil, stevia to nuts paste and transfer the mix to a saucepan
3. Stir cook for 5 minutes on high heat
4. Lower heat to low and simmer for 10 minutes
5. Serve warm and enjoy!

Nutrition (Per Serving)

- Calories: 260
- Fat: 22g
- Carbohydrates: 12g
- Protein: 6g

Chapter 5: Beef, Lamb, and Pork

Southern Pork Chops

Serving: 4
Prep Time: 2 minutes
Cook Time: 13 minutes

Ingredients

- Vegetable cooking oil spray
- 4 ounce of boneless pork loin chop trimmed off its fat
- 1/3 cup of salsa
- 2 tablespoon of fresh lime juice
- ¼ cup of fresh cilantro (chopped)

How To

1. Take a large-sized non-stick skillet and spray it with cooking spray
2. Heat it up until hot over high heat
3. Press the chops with your palm to flatten them slightly
4. Add them to the skillet and cook for 1 minute for each side until they are nicely browned
5. Lower down the heat to medium-low
6. Combine the salsa and lime juice
7. Pour the mix over the chops
8. Simmer uncovered for about 8 minutes until the chops are Perfectly done
9. If needed, sprinkle some cilantro on top
10. Serve!

Nutrition Values (Per Serving)

- Calories: 184
- Fat: 8g
- Carbohydrates: 2g
- Protein: 25g

Creamy Caramelized Onion Pork Chops

Prep Time: 10 minutes

Cooking Time: 30 minutes

Number of Servings: 2

Ingredients

- 4 pounds chuck roast
- 4 ounces green chile, chopped
- 2 tablespoons chili powder
- ½ teaspoon dried oregano
- ½ teaspoon ground cumin
- 2 garlic cloves, minced
- Salt as needed

How To

1. Rub the chops with a seasoning of 1 teaspoon of pepper and 2 teaspoons of salt
2. Take a skillet and place it over medium heat, add oil and allow the oil to heat up
3. Brown the seasoned chop both sides
4. Add water and onion to the skillet and cover, lower down the heat to low, and simmer for 20 minutes
5. Turn the chops over and season with more salt and pepper
6. Cover and cook until the water fully evaporates and the beef shows a slightly brown texture
7. Remove the chops and serve with a topping of the caramelized onion
8. Serve and enjoy!

Nutritional Values (Per Serving)

- Calories: 47
- Fat: 4 g
- Carbohydrates: 4 g
- Protein: 0.5g

Lamb and Mustard Cutlets

Prep Time: 10 minutes
Cooking Time: 10 minutes
Number of Servings: 2

Ingredients

- 1 tablespoon Dijon mustard
- 1 tablespoon honey
- 2 tablespoons white wine vinegar
- 15 ounces lamb cutlet, trimmed
- 1 and ½ cup brown rice, cooked
- 2 cups baby spinach leaves, shredded

How To

1. Take a small-sized bowl and add mustard, honey, vinegar, and mix well
2. Preheat your BBQ grill to high
3. Cook the cutlets for about 2 minutes Per side to ensure that they are cooked well
4. Brush half of your mustard mix near the end of the cooking
5. Take a microwave-safe bowl and add the rice, place them in your microwave, and cook
6. Stir in spinach leaves while the rice is hot
7. Divide the rice amongst your serving plates and top up with the grille cutlets
8. Drizzle the remaining mustard mix on top and enjoy!

Nutritional Values (Per Serving)

- Calories: 1507
- Fat: 124 g
- Saturated Fat: 26 g
- Carbohydrates: 55 g
- Fiber: 10 g
- Sodium: 370 mg
- Protein: 54 g

Subtle Herbed Beef Roast

Number of Servings: 3
Prep Time: 10 minutes
Cooking Time: 60-70 minutes

Ingredients

- 1-pound rump roast, boneless
- 1 tablespoon yellow mustard
- 1 teaspoon dried thyme
- ½ teaspoon dried rosemary
- 1 teaspoon dried parsley flakes
- Salt and pepper to taste
- ½ cup beef bone broth
- 4 garlic cloves, peeled and halved
- 2 yellow onions, quartered

How To

1. Pat your roast dry with a towel, rub roast with mustard spices all over
2. Place rump roast in roasting pan, pour beef broth
3. Scatter garlic and onions around meat, transfer to a pre-heated oven (360 degrees F)
4. Roast for 30 minutes, lower heat to 220 degrees F, roast for 30-40 minutes more
5. Serve and enjoy!

Nutritional Values (Per Serving)

- Calories: 316
- Fat: 13g
- Carbohydrates: 2g
- Protein: 47g

Purely Spanish Pork Cutlets and Onion

Prep Time: 10 minutes
Cooking Time: 10 minutes
Number of Servings: 4

Ingredients

- 1 tablespoon olive oil
- 2 pork cutlets
- 1 bell pepper, deveined and sliced
- 1 Spanish onion, chopped
- 2 garlic cloves, minced
- ½ teaspoon hot sauce
- ½ teaspoon mustard
- ½ teaspoon paprika
- Salt and pepper to taste

How To

1. Take a large saucepan, add olive oil and place it over medium-high heat
2. Let it heat up, add pork cutlets and fry for 3-4 minutes until golden and crispy on both sides
3. Lower temperature to medium and add bell pepper, Spanish onion, garlic, hot sauce, mustard and cook for 3 minutes until veggies are tender
4. Sprinkle paprika, salt, pepper and serve
5. Enjoy!

Nutritional Values (Per Serving)

- Calories: 24
- Fat: 3 g
- Saturated Fat: 1 g
- Carbohydrates: 2 g

Lovely Asian Beef Short Ribs

Serving: 4
Prep Time: 10 minutes
Cook Time: 10 minutes

Ingredients

- 2 pounds beef short ribs
- 1 tablespoon Szechuan peppercorns
- 2 tablespoons curry powder
- 6-piece star anise
- 1 onion, diced
- 3 tablespoons coconut aminos
- 1 tablespoon sesame oil
- 1 cup of water
- Salt and pepper, to taste

How To

1. Add all ingredients to the slow cooker and mix them well
2. Cook for 10 hours on low heat
3. Once done serve
4. Enjoy!

Nutrition Values (Per Serving)

- Calories: 442
- Fat: 26g
- Carbohydrates: 6g
- Protein: 47g

Chapter 6: Poultry

Lovely BBQ Slaw

Serving: 1
Prep Time: 5 minutes
Cook Time: 45 minutes

<u>Ingredients</u>

- 1 medium-sized raw Sweet Potato
- 1 medium skinless and raw chicken breast
- BBQ sauce as needed
- 1 tablespoon of low-fat Mayonnaise
- 1 tablespoon of natural Greek Yogurt
- 1 teaspoon of fresh lemon juice
- 1 and a ¾ ounce of finely shredded cabbage
- 1 ounce of grated raw carrots
- 1 medium spring onions finely sliced

<u>How To</u>

1. Pre: heat your oven to 352 degrees Fahrenheit
2. Prick the potato skin with a fork and place them on a baking tray, roast for 40:45 minutes
3. Take an ovenproof dish and add chicken and 2 tablespoons of water
4. Cover tightly with foil and bake for 25 minutes
5. Drain the cooking juice and cover the chicken with BBQ sauce
6. Turn well and coat it
7. Recover and bake for 15 minutes more
8. Take a bowl and add mayonnaise, yogurt, lemon juice, and season with black pepper
9. Stir in cabbage, spring onion, and carrot
10. Shred the chicken using 2 fork

11. Make a deep cut on top of the potato and top with chicken
12. Serve with the sale and enjoy it!

Nutrition Values (Per Serving)

- Calories: 472
- Fat: 26g
- Carbohydrates: 36g
- Protein: 24g

Mean Stir-Fried Chicken

Serving: 3
Prep Time: 10 minutes
Cook Time: 12 minutes

Ingredients

- 2 pieces(7 ounces each) chicken breast, skinless and boneless
- ¼ pound brown mushrooms
- 1 tablespoon virgin coconut oil
- ¼ onion, sliced thinly
- 1 large orange bell pepper
- 1 tablespoon soy sauce
- ¼ pound brown mushroom

How To

1. Take a nonstick saucepan and add heat coconut oil
2. Add soy sauce, mushrooms, chicken, and bell pepper
3. Stir fry for 8 to 10 minutes
4. Remove the pan and serve
5. Enjoy!

Nutrition Values (Per Serving)

- Calories: 227
- Fat: 2g
- Carbohydrates: 4g
- Protein: 32g

Epic Mango Chicken

Number of Servings: 4
Prep Time: 10 minutes
Cooking Time: 10 minutes

Ingredients

- 2 medium mangoes, peeled and sliced
- 10 ounces of coconut milk
- 4 teaspoons olive oil
- 4 teaspoons curry paste
- 14 ounces chicken breasts, skinless and boneless cut into cubes
- 4 medium shallots
- 1 large English cucumber, seeded and sliced

How To

1. Slice half of the mangoes and add the halves to a bowl
2. Add mangoes and coconut milk to a blender and blend until you have a smooth puree
3. Keep the mixture on the side
4. Take a large-sized pot and place it over medium heat, add oil and allow the oil to heat up
5. Add curry paste and cook for 1 minute until you have a nice fragrance; add shallots and chicken to the pot and cook for 5 minutes
6. Pour mango puree into the mix and allow it to heat up
7. Serve the cooked chicken with mango puree and cucumbers
8. Enjoy!

Nutritional Values (Per Serving)

- Calories: 400
- Fat: 20 g
- Carbohydrates: 31 g
- Protein: 26 g

Balsamic Chicken with Berry

Serving: 4
Prep Time: 10 minutes
Cook Time: 20 minutes

Ingredients

- 3 pieces of skinless and boneless chicken breast
- Salt as needed
- Black pepper as needed
- ¼ cup of all-purpose flour
- 2/3 cup of low-fat chicken broth
- 1 and a ½ teaspoon of corn starch
- ½ a cup of low sugar raspberry preserve
- 1 and a ½ tablespoon of balsamic vinegar

How To

1. Cut the chicken into bite-sized portions and season with salt and pepper
2. Dredge the meat into flour and shake off excess
3. Take a non-stick skillet and place it over medium heat
4. Add chicken and cook for 15 minutes, turning once halfway through
5. Remove cooked chicken and transfer to a plate
6. Add cornstarch, chicken broth, raspberry preserve into the skillet and stir in balsamic vinegar (keep the heat on medium)
7. Transfer the cooked chicken to the skillet
8. Cook for 15 minutes more, making sure to turn once
9. Serve and enjoy!

Nutrition Values (Per Serving)

- Calories: 546
- Fat: 35g
- Carbohydrates: 11g
- Protein: 44g

Spectacular Almond Chicken

Serving: 3
Prep Time: 15 minutes
Cook Time: 15 minutes

Ingredients

- 2 large chicken breast, boneless and skinless
- 1/3 cup lemon juice
- 1 and ½ cups seasoned almond meal
- 2 tablespoons coconut oil
- Lemon pepper, to taste
- Parsley for decoration

How To

1. Slice chicken breast in half
2. Pound out each half until ¼ inch thick
3. Take a pan and place it over medium heat, add oil and heat it up
4. Dip each chicken breast slice into lemon juice and let it sit for 2 minutes
5. Turnover and let the other side sit for 2 minutes as well
6. Transfer to almond meal and coat both sides
7. Add coated chicken to the oil and fry for 4 minutes Per side, making sure to sprinkle lemon pepper liberally
8. Transfer to a paper-lined sheet and repeat until all chicken is fried
9. Garnish with parsley and enjoy!

Nutrition Values (Per Serving)

- Calories: 325
- Fat: 24g
- Carbohydrates: 3g
- Protein: 16g

Lovely Chicken Salsa

Serving: 1
Prep Time: 4 minutes
Cook Time: 14 minutes

Ingredients

- 2 chicken breast
- 1 cup of salsa
- 1 taco seasoning mix
- 1 cup plain Greek Yogurt
- ½ a cup of kite ricotta/cashew cheese, cubed

How To

1. Take a skillet and place it over medium heat
2. Add chicken breast, ½ cup of salsa, and taco seasoning
3. Mix well and cook for 12-15 minutes until the chicken are done
4. Take the chicken out and cube them
5. Place the cubes on a toothpick and top with cheddar
6. Place yogurt and remaining salsa in cups and use as dips
7. Enjoy!

Nutrition Values (Per Serving)

- Calories: 359
- Fat: 14g
- Net Carbohydrates: 14g
- Protein: 43g

Clean Chicken Breast Salad

Serving: 4
Prep Time: 25 minutes
Cook Time: 30-55 minutes

Ingredients

- 3 and ½ ounces chicken breast
- 2 tablespoons spinach
- 1 and ¾ ounces lettuces
- 1 bell pepper
- 2 tablespoons olive oil
- Lemon juice to taste

How To

1. Boil chicken breast without adding salt cut the meat into small strips
2. Put the spinach in boiling water for a few minutes, cut into small strips
3. Cut pepper in strips as well
4. Add everything to a bowl and mix with juice and oil
5. Serve!

Nutrition Values (Per Serving)

- Calories: 100
- Fat: 11g
- Carbohydrates: 3g
- Protein: 6g

Chapter 7: Vegetarian

Nice and Cold Thai Salad

Serving: 4
Prep Time: 10 minutes
Cook Time: 25 minutes

<u>Ingredients</u>

- 2 small zucchini pieces
- 1 small cucumber
- 2 peeled and shredded carrots
- ½ a cup of mung bean sprouts
- ¼ cup of chopped cashews
- ¼ cup of chopped fresh cilantro
- ½ a cup of sunshine sauce

<u>For Sauce</u>

- ½ a cup of unsweetened sunflower seed butter
- ½ a cup of coconut milk
- 1 lime juiced
- 1 tablespoon of coconut aminos
- 1 minced garlic clove
- ½ a teaspoon of crushed red pepper flakes
- ½ a teaspoon of rice vinegar

<u>How To</u>

1. Add the sauce ingredients to a small bowl and mix
2. Peel the zucchini using peeler and julienne into long slices
3. Keep peeling until all four sides are peeled
4. Keep repeating the process with the remaining zucchini and cucumbers

5. Add the noodles to a medium mixing bowl and add shredded carrots, bean sprouts, chopped cashews, and cilantro
6. Allow it to chill for 30 minutes
7. Add a tablespoon of water to the sauce and take the sauce out
8. Pour it over salad and garnish with cilantro and cashews
9. Toss and enjoy it!

Nutrition Values (Per Serving)

- Calories: 187
- Fat: 12g
- Carbohydrates: 19g
- Protein: 4g

Turtle Friendly Premium Salad

Serving: 6
Prep Time: 5 minutes
Cook Time: 5 minutes

Ingredients

- 1 chopped up the heart of Romaine lettuce
- 3 diced Roma tomatoes
- 1 English dice cucumber
- 1 small-sized red onions
- ½ a cup of curly parsley, finely chopped up
- 2 tablespoon of virgin olive oil
- Juice of ½ a large lemon
- 1 teaspoon of garlic powder
- Salt as needed
- Pepper as needed

How To

1. Wash the vegetables thoroughly under cold water
2. Prepare them by chopping, dicing, or mincing as needed
3. Take a large salad bowl and transfer the prepped veggies
4. Add vegetable oil, olive oil, lemon juice, and spice
5. Toss well to coat
6. Serve chilled if preferred
7. Enjoy!

Nutrition Values (Per Serving)

- Calories: 200
- Fat: 8g
- Carbohydrates: 18g
- Protein: 10g

Almond and Blistered Beans

Serving: 4
Prep Time: 10 minutes
Cook Time: 20 minutes

Ingredients

- 1-pound fresh green beans end trimmed
- 1 and ½ tablespoon olive oil
- ¼ teaspoon sunflower seeds
- 1 and ½ tablespoons fresh dill, minced
- Juice of 1 lemon
- ¼ cup crushed almonds
- Sunflower seeds as needed

How To

1. Preheat your oven to 400-degree F
2. Add in the green beans with your olive oil and also with sunflower seeds
3. Then spread them in one single layer on a large-sized sheet pan
4. Roast it up for 10 minutes and stir it nicely, then roast for another 8-10 minutes
5. Remove it from the oven and keep stirring in the lemon juice alongside the dill
6. Top it up with crushed almonds and some flak sea sunflower seeds, and serve

Nutrition (Per Serving)

- Calories: 347
- Fat: 16g
- Carbohydrates: 6g
- Protein: 45g

Mouthwatering Garlic Tomatoes

Prep Time: 10 minutes

Cooking Time: 50 minutes

Number of Servings: 4

Ingredients

- ¼ cup olive oil
- Pepper and salt as needed
- 3 thyme sprigs, chopped
- 1 pound mixed cherry tomatoes
- 4 garlic cloves, crushed

How To

1. Take a nice baking dish, add tomatoes and drizzle olive oil on top
2. Sprinkle thyme
3. Season well with salt and pepper
4. Preheat your oven to 325 degrees F
5. Bake for 50 minutes
6. Serve and enjoy!

Nutritional Values (Per Serving)

- Calories: 100
- Fat: 0 g
- Saturated Fat: 0 g
- Carbohydrates: 1 g
- Protein: 6 g

Spanish Omelet

Prep Time: 10 minutes
Cooking Time: 5 minutes
Number of Servings: 4

Ingredients

- 1 teaspoon olive oil
- 2 whole eggs
- ½ cup baby spinach
- Salt to taste

How To

1. Take your blender and add eggs, spinach, pepper, salt, and blender until combined
2. Take a pan and place it over medium heat, add olive oil and let it heat up
3. Add egg mixture into the pan, cook for 2-3 minutes
4. Flip and cook for 2 minutes more
5. Enjoy!

Nutritional Values (Per Serving)

- Calories: 350
- Fat: 30 g
- Carbohydrates: 8 g
- Protein: 12 g

Heart-Felt BBQ Zucchini

Serving: 2
Prep Time: 10 minutes
Cook Time: 60 minutes

Ingredients

- Olive oil as needed
- 3 zucchinis
- ½ teaspoon black pepper
- ½ teaspoon mustard
- ½ teaspoon cumin
- 1 teaspoon paprika
- 1 teaspoon garlic powder
- 1 tablespoon of sea salt
- 1-2 stevia
- 1 tablespoon chili powder

How To

1. Preheat your oven to 300 degrees F
2. Take a small bowl and add cayenne, black pepper, salt, garlic, mustard, paprika, chili powder, and stevia
3. Mix well
4. Slice zucchini into 1/8 inch slices and mist them with olive oil
5. Sprinkle spice blend over zucchini and bake for 40 minutes
6. Remove and flip, mist with more olive oil and leftover spice
7. Bake for 20 minutes more
8. Serve!

Nutrition (Per Serving)

- Calories: 163
- Fat: 14g
- Carbohydrates: 3g
- Protein: 8g

Packed and Stuffed Bell Pepper

Serving: 2
Prep Time: 10 minutes
Cook Time: 10 minutes

Ingredients

- 4 bell peppers, halved and hollowed
- ½ cup quinoa, cooked
- 12 black olives, halved
- 1/3 cup tomatoes, sun-dried
- ½ cup baby spinach
- 2 garlic cloves, minced
- Salt and pepper for taste

How To

1. Preheat your oven to 400 degrees F
2. Take a bowl and add listed ingredients (except bell pepper), mix well
3. Bake for 10 minutes
4. Once done, stuff pepper with the quinoa mixture
5. Serve and enjoy!

Nutrition (Per Serving)

- Calories: 126
- Fat: 5g
- Carbohydrates: 19g
- Protein: 3g

Perfect Cauliflower Tabbouleh

Serving: 2
Prep Time: 10 minutes
Cook Time: Nil

Ingredients

- 4 cups cauliflower rice
- 1 and ½ cups cherry tomatoes quartered
- 3-4 tablespoons olive oil
- 1 cup parsley, fresh chopped
- 1 cup mint, fresh and chopped
- 1 cup snap peas, sliced thin
- 1 small cucumber, cut into ¼ inch pieces
- ¼ cup scallions, sliced thin
- 3-4 tablespoons lemon juice
- 1 teaspoon salt
- ½ teaspoon pepper

How To

1. Take a bowl and add cauliflower rice, tomatoes, mint, parsley, cucumber, scallions, snap peas and toss them well
2. Add olive oil, lemon juice and toss well
3. Season well with salt and pepper
4. Serve and enjoy!

Nutrition (Per Serving)

- Calories: 220
- Fat: 15g
- Carbohydrates: 20g
- Protein: 7g

Grilled Eggplant Steak Yums

Serving: 2

Prep Time: 10 minutes

Cook Time: 10 minutes

Ingredients

- 4 Roma tomatoes, diced
- 8 ounces cashew cream
- 2 eggplants
- 1 tablespoon olive oil
- 1 cup parsley, chopped
- 1 cucumber, diced
- Salt and pepper to taste

How To

1. Slice eggplants into three shtick steaks, drizzle with oil, season with salt and pepper
2. Grill in a pan for 4 minutes Per side
3. Top with remaining ingredients
4. Serve and enjoy!

Nutrition (Per Serving)

- Calories: 86
- Fat: 7g
- Carbohydrates: 12g
- Protein: 8g

Chapter 8: Soups and Stews

Generous Egg Drop Soup

Serving: 5
Prep Time: 5 minutes
Cook Time: 5 minutes

Ingredients

- 4 cups of low sodium chicken broth
- ½ a teaspoon of soy sauce
- ½ a cup of cooked, boneless, and skinless chopped up chicken breast
- ½ a cup of frozen green peas
- ¼ cup of thinly sliced green onion
- 1 lightly beaten eggs

How To

1. Take a saucepan and place it over medium heat; add chicken stock and soy sauce
2. Bring the mix to a boil and add peas, green onions, chicken, and stir
3. Bring the mix to boil once again
4. Remove the heat and slowly drizzle in the Egg
5. Wait for a minute until the egg sets in
6. Stir and ladle the soup into serving bowls
7. Enjoy!

Nutrition Values (Per Serving)

- Calories: 119
- Fat: 4g
- Carbohydrates: 8g
- Protein: 14g

Glorious Onion Soup

Serving: 4
Prep Time: 5 minutes
Cook Time: 25 minutes

<u>Ingredients</u>

- 2 large-sized finely sliced onion
- 2 cups of vegetable stock
- 1 teaspoon of brown sugar
- 1 cup of red wine
- 1 measure of brandy
- 1 teaspoon of herbs de Provence
- 4 slices of stale bread
- 4 ounce of strong grated cheese
- 1 ounce of grated parmesan
- 1 tablespoon of plain flour
- 2 tablespoon of olive oil
- 1 ounce of butter
- Salt as needed
- Pepper as needed

<u>How To</u>

1. Take a pan and place it over medium-high heat
2. Add oil and butter and allow it to heat up
3. Add onion and sugar and keep cooking until the sugar dissolves and the onions are slightly caramelized
4. Pour brandy and flambé and stir well to dish out flames
5. Add flour and herbs de Provence and stir
6. Add stock and followed by the gradual addition of the red wine
7. Season a bit and lower down the heat to low
8. Simmer for 20 minutes; add a bit more water if needed to make it less thick

9. Ladle the soup into bowls
10. Place rounds of stale bread on top and add a bit of cheese
11. Garnish with some parmesan
12. Broil for just a bit to melt the cheese, serve!

Nutritional Values (Per Serving)

- Calories: 55
- Fat: 1.7g
- Carbohydrates: 8g
- Protein: 3.6g

Spiced Up Chicken Vegetable Soup

Serving: 4
Prep Time: 10 minutes
Cook Time: 25 minutes

Ingredients

- 1-pound chicken, skinless
- 1 teaspoon basil, dried
- 1 small onion, diced
- 1 can tomatoes, diced
- 2 cups vegetable, frozen
- 3 bay leaves
- 1 garlic clove, minced
- 1 and ½ cups sweet potatoes, cubed
- ½ teaspoon red chili pepper flakes
- 1 jar spicy tomato sauce
- ½ teaspoon of sea salt
- 2 cups chicken broth

How To

1. Add all ingredients to your Dutch oven, mix them well
2. Season with salt and pepper
3. Simmer for 15 minutes
4. Then cook 10 minutes
5. Serve warm and enjoy!

Nutrition Values (Per Serving)

- Calories: 279
- Fat: 11g
- Carbohydrates: 18g
- Protein: 27g

Cajun Jambalaya Soup

Serving: 6
Prep Time: 15 minutes
Cook Time: 40 minutes

Ingredients

- 1-pound large shrimp, raw and deveined
- 4 ounces chicken, diced
- ¼ cup Frank's red-hot sauce
- 2 cups okra
- 3 tablespoons Cajun seasoning
- 2 bay leaves
- ½ head cauliflower
- 1 large can organic, diced
- 1 large onion, chopped
- 2 cloves garlic, diced
- 5 cups chicken stock
- 4 pepper

How To

1. Take a heavy-bottomed pot and add all ingredients except cauliflower
2. Place it over on high heat
3. Mix them well and bring it to boil
4. Once boiled, lower the heat to simmer
5. Simmer for 30 minutes
6. Rice the cauliflower in your blender
7. Stir into the pot and simmer for another 5 minutes
8. Serve and enjoy!

Nutrition Values (Per Serving)

- Calories: 143

- Fat: 3g
- Carbohydrates: 14g
- Protein: 18g

Homely Lobster Bisque

Serving: 4
Prep Time: 10 minutes
Cook Time: 6 minutes

Ingredients

- 1 cup of diced carrots
- 1 cup of diced celery
- 29 ounce of diced tomatoes
- 2 minced whole shallots
- 1 clove of minced garlic
- 1 tablespoon of butter
- 32-ounce chicken broth, low-sodium
- 1 teaspoon of dill, dried
- 1 teaspoon of freshly ground black pepper
- ½ a teaspoon of paprika
- 4 lobster tails
- 1 pint of heavy whipping cream

How To

1. Add butter, garlic, and minced shallots to a microwave-safe bowl
2. Microwave for 2-3 minutes on HIGH
3. Add tomatoes, celery, carrot, minced shallots, garlic to your Instant Pot
4. Add chicken broth and spices to the Pot
5. Use a knife to cut the lobster tails if you prefer and add them to the Instant Pot
6. Lock up the lid and cook on HIGH pressure for 4 minutes
7. Release the pressure naturally over 10 minutes
8. Use an immersion blender to puree to your desired chunkiness
9. Serve and enjoy!

Nutrition Values (Per Serving)

- Calories: 437
- Fats: 17g
- Carbs: 21g
- Protein: 38g

Chicken and Carrot Stew

Serving: 4
Prep Time: 15 minutes
Cook Time: 6 hours

Ingredients

- 4 boneless chicken breast, cubed
- 3 cups of carrots, peeled and cubed
- 1 cup onion, chopped
- 1 cup tomatoes, chopped
- 1 teaspoon of dried thyme
- 2 cups of chicken broth
- 2 garlic cloves, minced
- Salt and pepper as needed

Directions

1. Add all of the listed ingredients to a Slow Cooker
2. Stir and close the lid
3. Cook for 6 hours
4. Serve hot and enjoy!

Nutrition Values (Per Serving)

- Calories: 182
- Fat: 3g
- Carbohydrates: 10g
- Protein: 39g

Epic Thai Soup

Serving: 4
Prep Time: 10 minutes
Cook Time: 15 minutes

Ingredients

- 3 cups chicken stocks
- 1 tablespoon tom yum paste
- ½ garlic clove, chopped
- 3 stalks lemongrass, chopped
- 2 kaffir lime leaves
- 2 skinless and boneless chicken breast, shredded
- 4 ounces mushrooms, sliced
- 1 tablespoon fish sauce
- 1 tablespoon lime juice
- 1 teaspoon green chile pepper, chopped
- 1 bunch coriander, chopped
- 1 bunch coriander, chopped
- 1 sprig fresh basil, chopped

Directions

1. Take a large-sized saucepan and add chicken stock
2. Bring the mix to a boil
3. Stir in tom yum paste, garlic and cook for 2 minutes
4. Stir in lemongrass, kaffir lime leaves and simmer for 5 minutes over low heat
5. Add mushrooms, fish sauce, green chile, lime juice, pepper and keep cooking over medium heat until blended well
6. Remove the heat and serve warm with a garnish of coriander and basil
7. Enjoy!

Nutrition Values (Per Serving)

- Fat: 1.8g
- Protein: 10g
- Carbohydrate: 5g
- Calories: 71g

Chapter 9: Fish and Seafood

Juicy Cod Fingers Burger

Serving: 2
Prep Time: 15 minutes
Cook Time: 40 minutes

Ingredients

- 4 sprays of cooking spray
- 4 ounce of raw peeled parsnips
- 4 ounce of peeled raw carrots
- 1 medium sweet potato
- 1 medium raw egg whole, lightly beaten
- 8 ounce of raw cod
- 6 ounce of frozen peas
- 1 slice of lemon cut up into 4 wedges
- Chickpea shells/ bread crumbs for coating the fish

How To

1. Preheat your oven to 392 degrees Fahrenheit
2. Take 2 baking trays and mist with cooking spray
3. Cut parsnips, carrots, and sweet potatoes into chips
4. Transfer them to one cooking tray and mist with cooking spray
5. Roast for 40 minutes until golden, making sure to turn them halfway through
6. Crush the chickpea shells/bread crumbs with a rolling pin and transfer to a shallow dish
7. Put Egg in another shallow dish
8. Cut the cod in 8 thick fingers and dip them in the Egg and then in the crushed chickpeas/bread crumbs
9. Put the crumbled fish on the second tray and bake for 15 minutes
10. Cook the peas in a pan of boiling water for 4 minutes

11. Drain and serve with the fish fingers, lemon wedges, and chips

12. Enjoy!

<u>Nutrition Values (Per Serving)</u>

- Calories: 824
- Fat: 59g
- Carbohydrates: 22g
- Protein: 52g

Secret Recipe Used Shrimp Scampi

Serving: 4
Prep Time: 25 minutes
Cook Time: 0 minutes

Ingredients

- 4 teaspoon of olive oil
- 1 and a ¼ pound of medium shrimp
- 6-8 pieces of minced garlic cloves
- ½ a cup of low-sodium chicken broth
- ½ a cup of dry white wine
- ¼ cup of fresh lemon juice
- ¼ cup of fresh parsley + 1 tablespoon extra (all minced)
- ¼ teaspoon of salt
- ¼ teaspoon of freshly ground black pepper
- 4 slices of lemon

How To

1. Take a large-sized bowl and place it over medium-high heat
2. Add oil and allow the oil to heat up
3. Add shrimp and cook for 2-3 minutes
4. Add garlic and cook for 30 seconds
5. Take a slotted spoon and carefully transfer the cooked shrimp to your serving platter
6. Add broth, lemon juice, wine, ¼ cup of parsley, salt and pepper to the same skillet and bring the whole mix to a boil
7. Keep boiling until the sauce has been reduced to half
8. Spoon the sauce over the cooked shrimp
9. Garnish with a bit of parsley and lemon
10. Serve and enjoy!

Nutrition Values (Per Serving)

- Calories: 184
- Fat: 6g
- Carbohydrates: 6g
- Protein: 16g

Lovely Pistachio Fish

Serving: 4
Prep Time: 5 minutes
Cook Time: 10 minutes

Ingredients

- 4 (5 ounces) boneless sole fillets
- Sunflower seeds and pepper as needed
- ½ cup pistachios, finely chopped
- Juice of 1 lemon
- 1 teaspoon extra virgin olive oil

How To

1. Preheat your oven to 350 degrees Fahrenheit
2. Line a baking sheet with parchment paper and keep it on the side
3. Pat fish dry with kitchen towels and lightly season with sunflower seeds and pepper
4. Take a small bowl and stir in pistachios
5. Place sol on the prepped sheet and press 2 tablespoons of pistachio mixture on top of each fillet
6. Drizzle fish with lemon juice and olive oil
7. Bake for 10 minutes until the top is golden and fish flakes with a fork
8. Serve and enjoy!

Nutrition Values (Per Serving)

- Calories: 166
- Fat: 6g
- Carbohydrates: 2g
- Protein: 26g

Herbed Up Shrimp Risotto

Serving: 4
Prep Time: 10 minutes
Cook Time: 8 minutes

Ingredients

- 2 pound of shrimp with their tails removed
- 1 cup of instant rice
- 2 cups of vegetable broth
- 1 chopped up onion
- 1 cup of chicken breast cut into fine strips
- ¼ cup of lemon juice
- 1 teaspoon of crushed red pepper
- ¼ cup of parsley
- ¼ cup of fresh dill
- 6 pieces of chopped up garlic cloves
- 1 tablespoon of black pepper
- ½ a cup of parmesan
- 1 cup of cashew cheese

How To

1. Add the listed Ingredients to your Instant Pot and stir
2. Lock up the lid and cook on HIGH pressure for 8 minutes
3. Release the pressure naturally over 10 minutes
4. Open lid and top with cheese
5. Serve hot and enjoy!

Nutrition Values (Per Serving)

- Calories: 463
- Fat: 8g
- Carbohydrates: 63g
- Protein: 29g

Toasted Rye with Salmon and Avocado

Serving: 2
Prep Time: 10 minutes
Cook Time: 0 minutes

Ingredients

- ½ of a medium avocados
- 1 tablespoon of chopped fresh chives
- 2 teaspoon of lime juice
- ½ a teaspoon of chili flakes
- ½ teaspoon of chili flakes
- 2 slices of dark rye bread
- 1 medium fresh Lebanese cucumber (thinly sliced)
- 5 ounce of smoked salmon
- 1 ounce of trimmed snow peas

How To

1. Take a small-sized bowl and add avocados, chives, chili, and juice
2. Take a fork and mash everything until you have a smooth mixture
3. Season with some freshly ground black pepper and salt
4. Toast your bread carefully to ensure that you don't burn them
5. Spread the avocado mix over the toast and serve with some cucumber, salmon, pea shoot
6. Enjoy!

Nutrition Values (Per Serving)

- Calories: 194
- Fat: 19g
- Carbohydrates: 4g
- Protein: 3g

Scrambled Eggs and Shrimp

Prep Time: 10 minutes
Cooking Time: 20 minutes
Number of Servings: 4

Ingredients:

- 1 tablespoon olive oil
- 1 onion, chopped
- 6 eggs, beaten
- 1 teaspoon salt
- 10 large shrimp, cooked
- ¼ cup cocktail sauce

Method:

1. Take a large-sized skillet and place it over medium heat
2. Add onion and Sauté for 5-10 minutes until translucent
3. Add eggs into the onion, add salt, and season
4. Cook for 5 minutes and stir until the eggs are set
5. Mix in cocktail sauce, shrimp into the eggs
6. Cook for 3-4 minutes
7. Once the mixture is warm
8. Serve and enjoy!

Nutritional Values (Per Serving)

- Calories: 236
- Fat: 14 g
- Carbohydrates: 8 g
- Protein: 16 g

Delicious Calamari Chili

Prep Time: 10 minutes + 1-hour marinating time
Cooking Time: 8 minutes
Number of Servings: 3

Ingredients:

- 2 tablespoons red bell pepper, minced
- 2 tablespoons, cilantro, chopped
- 1 and ½ pound squid cleaned and split open, tentacles cut into ½ inch rounds
- Dash of salt
- 1 lime, juiced
- 1 lime, zest
- ½ teaspoon ground cumin
- 1 teaspoon chili powder
- 2 tablespoons extra virgin olive oil

Method:

1. Take a medium-sized bowl, add olive oil, chili powder, cumin, zest, salt, juice, and pepper
2. Add squid to the mix, coat well with the marinade
3. Let it chill for 1 hour in your fridge
4. Set your oven to broil mode
5. Arrange squid on a baking sheet, broiled in your oven for 8 minutes, making sure to turn them once
6. Once tender, garnish the broiled calamari with red bell pepper and cilantro
7. Enjoy!

Nutritional Values (Per Serving)

- Calories: 156
- Fat: 13 g
- Carbohydrates: 12 g
- Protein: 3 g

Crunchy Hazelnut Sea Bass

Prep Time: 10 minutes

Cooking Time: 15 minutes

Number of Servings: 4

Ingredients:

- ½ cup hazelnuts, roasted
- 2 sea bass fillets
- ¼ teaspoon cayenne pepper
- 2 tablespoons clarified butter

Method:

1. Preheat your oven to 425 degrees F
2. Take a baking dish and line with parchment paper
3. Melt butter in a pan and brush it over the fish
4. Take a food processor and add the remaining ingredients
5. Coat sea bass with the hazelnut mix
6. Transfer to oven and bake for 15 minutes until fully cooked
7. Enjoy!

Nutritional Values (Per Serving)

- Calories: 336
- Fat: 29 g
- Carbohydrates: 05.5 g
- Protein: 16 g

Broccoli and Tilapia

Serving: 2

Prep Time: 4 minutes

Cook Time: 14 minutes

Ingredients

- 6 ounce of tilapia, frozen
- 1 tablespoon of almond butter
- 1 tablespoon of garlic, minced
- 1 teaspoon of lemon pepper seasoning
- 1 cup of broccoli florets, fresh

How To

1. Preheat your oven to 350 degrees Fahrenheit.
2. Add fish in aluminum foil packets.
3. Arrange broccoli around fish.
4. Sprinkle lemon pepper on top.
5. Close the packets and seal.
6. Bake for 14 minutes.
7. Take a bowl and add garlic and almond butter, mix well, and keep the mixture on the side.
8. Remove the packet from the oven and transfer to a platter.
9. Place almond butter on top of the fish and broccoli, serve and enjoy!

Nutrition Values (Per Serving)

- Calories: 362
- Fat: 25g
- Net Carbohydrates: 2g
- Protein: 29g

Spicer Lover's Baked Cod

Serving: 5
Prep Time: 15 minutes
Cook Time: 15 minutes

Ingredients

- 5 cod fillets
- 2 tablespoons curry powder
- 2 tablespoons olive oil
- 2 tablespoons plain Yogurt, non-fat
- 1 teaspoon ginger, grated
- 1 teaspoon soy sauce
- 2 and ½ teaspoon cayenne pepper
- 1 teaspoon of rice wine vinegar

How To

1. Preheat your oven to 400-degree F
2. Take a shallow dish, add all ingredients except oil
3. Mix well and let it marinate for 1 hour
4. Once ready, grease cookie sheet with oil
5. Place cod fillet on a prepared cookie sheet
6. Bake for 15 minutes
7. Serve and enjoy!

Nutrition Values (Per Serving)

- Calories: 254
- Fat: 1g
- Carbohydrates: 2g
- Protein: 42g

Supreme Lemon and Pepper Salmon

Serving: 4
Prep Time: 10 minutes
Cook Time: 20 minutes

Ingredients

- 4 salmon fillets
- 2 tablespoons olive oil
- 1 teaspoon lemon juice
- 2 tablespoons soy sauce
- Salt and pepper, to taste

How To

1. Place a trivet or steamer basket inside your pot
2. Pour water up to an inch high
3. Bring it to boil
4. Place the salmon fillets in a baking dish that fit
5. Put the rest of the ingredients and mix them well
6. Cover the dish securely with foil
7. Place the baking dish on the steam rack
8. Close the lid properly and steam for 15 minutes
9. Turn off the fire and wait for 5 minutes more.
10. Once done, it is ready to serve
11. Enjoy!

Nutrition Values (Per Serving)

- Calories: 239
- Fat: 16g
- Carbohydrates: 0.9g
- Protein: 20.2g

Hearty Tuna Salad

Serving: 4

Prep Time: 10 minutes

Cook Time: Nil

Ingredients

- 12 ounces white tuna, in water
- ½ cup celery, diced
- 2 tablespoons fresh parsley, chopped
- 2 tablespoons low-calorie Mayonnaise
- ½ teaspoon Dijon mustard
- ½ teaspoon salt
- ¼ teaspoon fresh ground black pepper

Direction

1. Take a medium-sized bowl and add tuna, parsley, and celery
2. Mix well and add Mayonnaise
3. Season with pepper and salt
4. Stir and add olives, relish, chopped pickle, onion and mix well
5. Serve and enjoy

Nutrition Values (Per Serving)

- Calories: 137
- Fat: 5g
- Carbohydrates: 1g
- Protein: 20g

Chapter 10: Desserts and Beverages

Delicious Carrot Cake

Serving: 4
Prep Time: 10 minutes
Cook Time: 0 minutes

Ingredients

- ¾ cup of all-purpose flour
- ½ a cup of yellow cornmeal
- 1 and a ½ teaspoon of baking powder
- ½ a teaspoon of ground cinnamon
- ¼ teaspoon salt
- ½ a cup of thawed frozen apple juice concentrate
- ¼ cup of fat-free milk
- 4 tablespoon of canola oil
- 1 large egg
- 2 tablespoon of brown sugar
- 1 cup of shredded carrots
- ½ a cup of raisin

For frosting

- ½ a cup of light cream cheese
- 1 tablespoon of honey

How To

1. Preheat your oven to 375 degrees Fahrenheit
2. Spray a 9 inch Bundt pan with cooking spray
3. Take a bowl and whisk in flour, cornmeal, baking powder, salt, and cinnamon
4. Use an electric mixer to beat apple juice concentrate, milk, oil, Egg, brown sugar in a large bowl

5. Beat in carrots and raisins and reduce the mixer speed
6. Add flour mixture and keep beating until blended well
7. Scrape the mixture into your pan
8. Bake for 35:40 minutes and check using a toothpick; it should come out clean
9. Combine cream cheese and honey in a food processor
10. Invert the cake onto a plate and use a narrow spatula to spread the frosting over the cake
11. Enjoy!

Nutrition Values (Per Serving)

- Calories: 155
- Fat: 1g
- Carbohydrates: 15g
- Protein: 3g

Elixir of Life

Serving: 2
Prep Time: 5 minutes
Cook Time: nil

Ingredients

- 15 leaves beet greens
- 1 beetroot, 3-inch diameter
- 7 medium carrots, diced
- 2 kale leaves, 8-12 inches sized

How To

1. Add the ingredients to your juicer or centrifuge
2. Process them thoroughly until you have a smooth juice
3. Pour the drink into a glass and give it a nice shake
4. Chill if you want and serve!

Nutrition (Per Serving)

- Calories: 177
- Fat: 1.79g
- Carbohydrates: 58g
- Protein: 14g

Strawberry and Melon Medley

Serving: 2
Prep Time: 5 minutes
Cook Time: nil

Ingredients

- 1 medium apple, cubed
- 1 orange fruit
- 1 whole cut strawberry
- 1 whole cup watermelon, diced

How To

1. Add the ingredients to your juicer or centrifuge
2. Process them thoroughly until you have a smooth juice
3. Pour the drink into a glass and give it a nice shake
4. Chill if you want and serve!

Nutrition (Per Serving)

- Calories: 144
- Fat:0.78g
- Carbohydrates: 43g
- Protein: 2.45g

Hearty Rice Pudding

Serving: 4

Prep Time: 10 minutes

Cook Time: 20-30 minutes

Ingredients

- 1 cup of brown rice
- 1 teaspoon vanilla extract
- ½ teaspoon salt
- ½ teaspoon cinnamon
- ¼ teaspoon nutmeg
- 3 egg substitute
- 3 cups coconut milk, light
- 2 cups brown rice, cooked

How To

1. Take a bowl and mix in all ingredients, stir well
2. Preheat your oven to 300 degrees F
3. Transfer mixture to a baking dish and transfer dish to the oven
4. Bake for 90 minutes
5. Serve and enjoy!

Nutrition (Per Serving)

- Calories: 330
- Fat: 10g
- Carbohydrates: 52g
- Protein: 5g

Sublime Oatmeal Cookies

Serving: 4
Prep Time: 10 minutes
Cook Time: 15 minutes

Ingredients

- 1/4 cup applesauce
- 1/2 teaspoon cinnamon
- 1/3 cup raisins
- 1/2 teaspoon vanilla extract, pure
- 1 cup ripe banana, mashed
- 2 cups oatmeal

How To

1. Preheat your oven to 350 degrees F
2. Take a bowl and mix in everything until you have a gooey mixture
3. Pour batter into ungreased baking sheet drop by drop and flatten them using a tablespoon
4. Transfer to your oven, bake for 15 minutes
5. Serve once ready!

Nutrition (Per Serving)

- Calories: 80
- Fat: 1g
- Carbohydrates: 16g
- Protein: 2g

Healthy Chocolate Coconut Bars

Serving: 16 bars
Prep Time: 20 minutes + 20 minutes chill time
Cook Time: Nil

Ingredients

- ¼ cup coconut oil,
- 2 cups unsweetened shredded coconut
- ¼ cup of sugar
- 2 tablespoons pure maple syrup
- 1 cup vegan chocolate chips

How To

1. Coat 8-inch square baking dish with parchment paper, take a small bowl and add coconut, sugar, maple syrup, coconut oil
2. Transfer mixture to baking dish and press firmly
3. Take a small microwave-safe bowl and heat chocolate chips on high for 1 minute
4. Stir and heat until the chocolate has completely melted in intervals of 30 seconds
5. Pour melted chocolate over coconut base, let it chill for 20 minutes
6. Once done, serve and enjoy!

Nutrition (Per Serving)

- Calories: 305
- Fat: 20g
- Carbohydrates: 19g
- Protein: 3g

Cinnamon and Pumpkin Fudge

Serving: 4
Prep Time: 5 minutes + 20 minutes chill time
Cook Time: Nil

Ingredients

- 1 teaspoon ground cinnamon
- 1 cup pumpkin puree
- ¼ teaspoon nutmeg, ground
- 1 and ¾ cup of coconut butter, melted
- 1 tablespoon coconut oil

How To

1. Take a bowl and mix in pumpkin spices, coconut butter, coconut oil and whisk well
2. Spread mixture into pan and cover with foil, press it down well
3. Discard the foil
4. Let it chill for 2 hours
5. Chop into squares, serve and enjoy!

Nutrition (Per Serving)

- Calories: 110
- Fat: 10g
- Carbohydrates: 5g
- Protein: 1.2g

Chia Pudding with Zucchini

Serving: 4
Prep Time: 70 minutes
Cook Time: Nil

Ingredients

- 1 whole mango, peeled and pureed
- 1 whole cup of coconut milk
- 3 tablespoons chia seeds

How To

1. Add the listed ingredients to a bowl and stir
2. Let it chill for 60 minutes
3. Serve and enjoy!

Nutrition (Per Serving)

- Calories: 146
- Fat: 26g
- Carbohydrates: 15g
- Protein: 23g

Amazing Mango and Chia Puddings

Prep Time: 70 minutes
Cooking Time: Nil
Number of Servings: 4

Ingredients:

- 1 whole mango, peeled and pureed
- 1 whole cup of coconut milk
- 3 tablespoons chia seeds

Method:

1. Add listed ingredients to a bowl and stir well
2. Let it chill for 60 minutes
3. Serve and enjoy!

Nutritional Values (Per Serving)

- Calories: 136
- Fat:3 g
- Saturated Fat: 1 g
- Carbohydrates: 0.9 g
- Protein: 24 g

Trail Mix

Prep Time: 10 minutes
Cooking Time: 55 minutes
Number of Servings: 4

Ingredients:

- ¼ cup raw cashew
- Salt as needed
- 2 tablespoons melted coconut oil
- 1 teaspoon cinnamon
- ¼ cup walnuts
- ¼ cup almonds
- ¼ cup raw cashews

How To

1. Take a baking sheet and carefully line it with parchment paper
2. Preheat your oven to 275 degrees F
3. Take a bowl and melt coconut oil; take another large-sized bowl
4. Add nuts to the bowl, cinnamon, and coconut oil
5. Stir well. Season with salt
6. Transfer bowl to your oven
7. Bake for 6 minutes until brown
8. Enjoy!

Nutritional Values (Per Serving)

- Calories: 363
- Fat:22 g
- Carbohydrates: 41 g
- Protein: 7 g

Awesome Oat Bars

Prep Time: 10 minutes

Cooking Time: 30 minutes

Number of Servings: 6

Ingredients

- 2 cups oats
- Non-stick spray
- 1 cup unsweetened coconut, shredded
- ½ teaspoon salt
- ¼ cup raw turbinado sugar
- ¼ cup flaxseed
- ¼ cup toasted sesame seeds
- 2 tablespoons psyllium powder
- ¾ cup butter
- ¼ cup honey

How To

1. Preheat your oven to 350 degrees F
2. Take an 11x7 cake pan and grease well
3. Take a large-sized bowl and add oats, coconut, salt, sugar, flaxseed, psyllium, and sesame
4. Take a small pan and place it over low heat
5. Add butter and honey, let it melt
6. Add the honey mix to the bowl with dry ingredients
7. Mix well
8. Transfer to prepared baking pan and press them firmly into a fine layer
9. Bake for 25 minutes, remove and cut into 9 bars
10. Serve and enjoy!

Nutritional Values (Per Serving)

- Calories: 365
- Fat: 14 g
- Carbohydrates: 55 g
- Protein: 9 g

Lovely Zucchini Brownies

Serving: 4
Prep Time: 5 minutes
Cook Time: 30-45 minutes

Ingredients

- 2 cups flour
- 1 and ½ cups vegan sugar
- 1 teaspoon baking soda
- 1 teaspoon salt
- ½ cup cocoa, unsweetened
- 2 tablespoons vanilla extract
- ½ cup oil
- 2 cups zucchini, peeled and grated

How To

1. Take a bowl and sift in cocoa, salt, flour, sugar, and baking soda
2. Stir well
3. Add oil, vanilla, zucchini mix well until you have a nice batter
4. Transfer to a baking dish, preheat your oven to 350 degrees F
5. Pour mixture baking dish, transfer to the oven
6. Bake for 30-45 minutes until done

Nutrition (Per Serving)

- Calories: 138
- Fat: 5g
- Carbohydrates: 21g
- Protein: 1.5g

Premium Blue Drink

Serving: 2
Prep Time: 5 minutes
Cook Time: nil

Ingredients

- 1 medium apple, 3-inch diameter
- 1 broccoli stalk, diced
- 6 large carrots, diced
- 1 medium whole tomato, diced
- ½ cup blueberries

How To

1. Add the ingredients to your juicer or centrifuge
2. Process them thoroughly until you have a smooth juice
3. Pour the drink into a glass and give it a nice shake
4. Chill if you want and serve!

Nutrition (Per Serving)

- Calories: 233
- Fat: 1.8g
- Carbohydrates: 70g
- Protein: 7g

Weight Loss Booster

Serving: 2
Prep Time: 5 minutes
Cook Time: nil

Ingredients

- 7 medium carrots
- ½ a lemon fruit
- 7 peppermint leaves
- ½ a pineapple fruit

How To

1. Add the ingredients to your juicer or centrifuge
2. Process them thoroughly until you have a smooth juice
3. Pour the drink into a glass and give it a nice shake
4. Chill if you want and serve!

Nutrition (Per Serving)

- Calories: 235
- Fat: 10g
- Carbohydrates: 71g
- Protein: 4g

Beautiful Banana Custard

Serving: 3
Prep Time: 10 minutes
Cook Time: 25 minutes

Ingredients

- 2 ripe bananas, peeled and mashed finely
- ½ a teaspoon of vanilla extract
- 14-ounce unsweetened almond milk
- 3 eggs

Directions

1. Preheat your oven to 350 degrees Fahrenheit
2. Grease 8 custard glasses lightly
3. Arrange the glasses in a large baking dish
4. Take a large bowl and mix all of the ingredients and mix them well until combined nicely
5. Divide the mixture evenly between the glasses
6. Pour water into the baking dish
7. Bake for 25 minutes
8. Take it out and serve
9. Enjoy!

Nutrition Values (Per Serving)

- Calories: 59
- Fat: 2.4g
- Carbohydrates: 7g
- Protein: 3g

Gentle Blackberry Crumble

Serving: 4
Prep Time: 10 minutes
Cook Time: 45 minutes
Smart Points: 4

Ingredients

- ½ a cup of coconut flour
- ½ a cup of banana, peeled and mashed
- 6 tablespoon of water
- 3 cups of fresh blackberries
- ½ a cup of arrowroot flour
- 1 and a ½ teaspoon of baking soda
- 4 tablespoon of butter, melted
- 1 tablespoon of fresh lemon juice

Directions

1. Preheat your oven to 300 degrees F
2. Take a baking dish and grease it lightly
3. Take a bowl and mix all of the ingredients except blackberries; mix well
4. Place blackberries in the bottom of your baking dish and top with flour
5. Bake for 40 minutes
6. Serve and enjoy!

Nutrition Values (Per Serving)

- Calories: 12
- Fat: 7g
- Carbohydrates: 10g
- Protein: 4g

Conclusion

I can't express how honored I am to think that you found my book interesting and informative enough to read it all through to the end.

I thank you again for purchasing this book, and I hope you had as much fun reading it as I had writing it.

I bid you farewell and encourage you to move forward with your amazing weight watchers journey!